I0116129

SAVE YOUR LIFE PREVENT HOSPITAL USE

PHILOSOPHY OF ACTION DESIGN AND MULTIPLICITY

BOOK 3

DAN PAUL

PROACT 2525

Copyright © 2024 by Dan Paul

All rights reserved.

No part of this book may be reproduced in any form or by any electronic or mechanical means, including information storage and retrieval systems, without written permission from the author, except for the use of brief quotations in a book review.

❀ Created with Vellum

CONTENTS

1. Prevention   1
2. Balancing Risk and Danger   9
3. Strategies to Minimize Risk   18
4. Building Performance   24
5. Awareness To Avoid Injury   34
6. Goals and Habits   38
7. Growing a Care Team   44
8. Insurance   50
9. Herbs   60
10. Hospital Strategies   68

About the Author   71
Also by Dan Paul   73

CHAPTER 1
PREVENTION

Prevention

Preventing hospital use generates benefits that last a lifetime. Developing routines that build up your body's strength, resilience, and immunity is empowering. As you grow your muscle power, eat well, and set your mind to avoid unsafe living, your awareness and enjoyment of life will increase. Hospital visits can save your life but also compromise your ability to live. Caution, research, and help from others can increase your chances of staying out of the hospital. If you get medical help, a care team can help avoid preventable accidents and infections.

Build Your Body

Bodies come alive as they move, and die when they stop. Developing goals and routines can help you stay fit, happy, and out of the hospital. Exercise and muscle building can make you able to withstand stresses that put people in bed or on the couch for extended periods. By making attainable goals, you can measure and track your performance. With care and diligence, you can develop habits that make exercising and muscle-building a routine that adds strength, confidence, and willpower to your life. As you increase the strength of your body, you can develop a mindset that steers clear of accidents, bad habits, and mediocre health care.

Build Your Mind

Of course, your mind is a terrible thing to waste. With attention and vision, you can move through the snares that catapult you into a hospital. Foresight, research, and planning can set your mind to minimize accidents. Meditation reduces stress, increases oxygen in your brain, and helps you relax so you can think and make decisions. Being safe may require staying one step ahead of the people you interact with. Accidents happen in a split second. Peak alertness, reflexes, and coordination can give you the advantage that keeps you healthy, active, and wise.

Stress

Stress is good and bad. Without a challenge, boredom and depression creep in. Stress impedes action and desire. Letting go dissolves stress. Fun sports, horsing around with kids, playing your favorite games, sex, and other activities can dissolve stress. Meditation and marijuana melt stress. When you find an activity that gets you so involved that you lose track of time, space, and appointments, you have another tool to erase nagging thoughts that undermine your ability to act.

Cultivating Motivation

Cultivating motivation is a fine art. Creating the conditions for inspired output requires effort, practice, and ingenuity. Starting with your body may yield significant gains. Set goals and stay on target by developing exercise habits. Eat at least two servings of fresh produce each meal, and consider eating just enough to get you to your next meal. Use power herbs like ginseng, marijuana, and sarsaparilla root to get your motor running. Practice meditating while waiting for people, in transit, and as time affords. Design your goals to include fuel for motivation. Look for inspiration from children, people, plants and animals. Practice positive relationships with all the people you interact with. If you can practice achieving the challenges in this book, you won't have problems with motivation.

Cultivating Power

Motivation requires energy. From inside, the energy flows out. Eat ginseng and let it work magic. Cultivate energy to make power. Food is a source of energy. Exercise is energy. To make power, combine food, exercise, and mindset. These forces lead people to take on and finish big projects. Power is the ability to work and complete projects. Power is the output of your body, nutrition, and exercise that builds strength. Your mind is a muscle; push it to build strength. For some, power is the ability to meet needs and wants sustainably. As you grow your life force, your energy will inspire you.

Importance of Communication

Communicating effectively with your doctor is crucial. Leaving out information may lead to the wrong diagnosis. Hopefully, a doctor has enough time to ask enough questions and observe your behavior. Many are under a lot of pressure to see patients quickly. Paperwork, difficult patients, and lawsuits take a toll on doctors. Understanding what your doctor is saying can also be an issue. After frequently rifling off so many instructions to patients, a doctor may not realize that a patient will not understand the instructions without a slow and careful explanation of the diagnosis and treatment. A diagnosis is based on the information you provide, a doctor's observations and interpretations of x-rays, test results, and data. The results must be analyzed and interpreted correctly. With so many variables in the equation, it's essential to think through the process carefully and to ask people you trust if everything makes sense.

Patient Quagmire: A patient must evaluate a doctor but needs to gain the skills and knowledge of a doctor.

As a patient, you are under the care of your doctor. The doctor controls how medicine is administered. The physician has specialized knowledge and decides what your problem is and how to fix it. If the diagnosis is wrong, it's likely that the solution will not work. So, a patient should evaluate the doctor to make sure they diagnose and prescribe the right medical solution. Before you see a doctor, write down or speak about your problem so that you can communicate well. Try to answer the question out loud and by writing it out. Then do research and ask more questions to yourself and to anyone who will listen. Write down the best answer you come up with, then try to figure out what's wrong with your answer. Write that down and do more research. Continue the process of investigation as long as you can. Ideally you would have trusted doctors to talk to, but that's often not the case. A patient's dilemma is that they must evaluate the diagnosis and solution, yet may need to be qualified to do so. Write down your questions for the doctor. You must ask essential and challenging questions. If the doctor doesn't seem to listen, ask for an explanation. If you still don't get the desired results, it's time to look for and use another doctor. Choosing a doctor you can trust makes a big difference. With a team of people to help, you can generate better solutions.

Stakes are High

It's your body, take it seriously. With significant effort, you will stay healthy. You must avoid processed foods that taste great but could be a ticking time bomb in your body. You must evaluate the diagnosis and solution of your doctor. Does it include all of the symptoms? Do the complications and side effects from the treatment outweigh the benefits? You can get a second opinion, but this may take time and money, which many people don't have. If you develop a relationship with another doctor before all this happens, you will be in a better position to make a decision. Going to the hospital carries many risks that people may need to be aware of. Hospitals must follow laws that may not seem in your interest. Researching what is going on in your body may provide essential results.

Care Team

A care team can help you stay well and help you avoid preventable mistakes and deadly infections in the hospital. It could be family, friends, or people with similar health issues. Growing a care team can add stability and security to your life. Relatives and friends are often the best places to start. When you trust and like someone, it's more likely that you can work together on a care team. When the care load is shared, it's easier. One person caring for someone who needs a lot of help is quite challenging. Cultivating communities of mutual aid could make a difference, especially when you have no family and few friends. Getting organized can make a big difference. People who live close are a good option since they can quickly come and go without a lot of travel. A care team can help you get to and from appointments, get food and medicine, research and review doctor's suggestions, and be at the hospital when needed. Patients who have someone at the hospital watching what is going on have a better chance of getting good care.

Family Medical History

If you have relatives, it helps to learn what illnesses run in the family. When heart disease, cancer, and diabetes undermine multiple members of a family, it may indicate that a genetic component is active. Behavior is easier to change than genes. Many common illnesses can be prevented by changing your diet, exercising, and reducing stress. When you know three family members have died from heart disease, be sure to tell your doctor.

Knowing Your Body is Crucial

Do I need to see a doctor? Often, it's hard to know. If you can get better without help, that can be good, but not if you make something worse. Exercising to make your body strong helps a lot. It's a way to prevent problems. Boosting your immunity is another great skill to keep healthy and out of the hospital. As you go through an illness, taking notes about what happens, about what works and doesn't work, can help in the future. Often, the same problems occur over and over. With your medical log, you can track what is going on with your body over the long term. Reviewing the log reminds you of what happened and may have a solution.

Personal Medical Log

A medical log increases your ability to stay healthy and out of the hospital. Keeping track of what works and what doesn't can provide important shortcuts to staying well. Often, we have recurring problems. A common one is back problems, especially for people who lift a lot, carry weight, or do manual labor. For most people, if they aren't strengthening their abdomen muscles regularly, they will always have back problems. With a log, you can track what works and what doesn't. People are creatures of habit. They learn and avoid things. They understand and repeat what works. It's easy to fall into bad habits. With motivation, you can prevent that. A medical log is a journal. A standard format with dates, length of illness, diagnosis, research, solutions tried, solutions failed and solutions that worked can be a good place to start.

Using a Spreadsheet

Keeping track of your health could be done as a spreadsheet and a standard writing program. Keeping information in one format can make it easy to find later. A spreadsheet may work well. Columns could include sickness, the start date, and when it was over. What didn't work, What did work, and Which person helped the most? Which websites were most relevant? As you go along, you can develop more columns to include. Often, the challenge is to record what is happening. Spreadsheets can help you focus on what matters most and help you avoid forgetting something. Spreadsheets help track information, make standard formats, stay organized, and recognize patterns to help you stay out of the hospital.

Needles, Doctors, Hospitals Fear and Loathing

Some people are afraid of needles, others are afraid of doctors, while others avoid the hospital altogether. This avoidance may keep you alive but may catch up to you. At some point, you may have to go to the hospital. If you get checkups regularly, it's less effort than if you never go to the hospital. A lot depends on what you do. Even if you eat well, exercise, and minimize your stress, you could die from someone else's mistake. Generally, you have better odds if you take good care of yourself.

Can I get in? If I get in, will I become an indentured servant?

Many people believe the United States has the best healthcare system in the world, but is it perfect if you can't use it? Or, if you get in but must work forever to pay it back? And once you get in, what are the dangers of the system? If you make a lot of money, the healthcare system is affordable. Many others find a way to get into the system; others have just enough access, and some only use the emergency room. Others do everything possible to avoid going to a hospital. Avoiding hospital visits requires design, effort, and discipline.

Education System

Children learn bits and pieces of healthcare information in public and private schools nationwide. Rarely is there a deeper focus on how to live strong and healthy in ways that generate a pleasant, active, and pain-free life. A wealth of information is available for people with internet access, but for many, it's a question of motivation. Still, with higher standards, better curriculum, and leadership at many levels, another curriculum could empower students to have a more positive, active, and beneficial life. Preventing problems is often easier than fixing them later. With goals, schools can help students live healthy, active lives free of accidents and medical problems.

Prevention

If this book is about one word, it's prevention. Preventing what? Accidents and illness kill many people; if you can avoid accidents while developing healthy habits, your chances of living well are better. Does your doctor help you prevent illness? Many doctors can't because they have so many other things to do; some choose not to, and a few doctors prevent illness by guiding patients into healthy habits.

Prevent a Stroke http://www.health.harvard.edu/womens-health/8-things-you-can-do-to-prevent-a-stroke

Lower your blood pressure

Loose weight

Exercise in moderation

One glass of alcohol per day

Treat irregular heartbeat

Treat diabetes

Quit smoking

Identify a stroke fast Face, Arms, Speech, Time

Prevent Heart disease http://www.mayoclinic.org/diseases-conditions/heart-disease/basics/prevention/con-20034056

Certain types of heart disease, such as heart defects, can't be prevented. However, other types of heart disease may be prevented or minimized by doing the following:

• Quit smoking

• Control other health conditions, such as high blood pressure, high cholesterol and diabetes

• Do aerobic exercises 3-4 times per week

• Eat a low salt and low saturated fat food diet

• Maintain a healthy weight

• Reduce and manage stress

• Practice good hygiene

Prevent or minimize diabetes by doing the following: CBECSSE

Control blood sugar
Be active for 30 minutes a day
Eat heart-healthy food
Check your blood pressure
Shred pounds if you are overweight
Stop smoking
Eat well 2-3 servings of fruits and vegetables per meal

CHAPTER 2
BALANCING RISK AND DANGER

Tricky Risk

Risk is tricky. We move toward it and away from it at the same time. Enveloped in risk, we throw the dice and make our way through the world. With our risk tolerances, we live in areas of danger. We move toward some and away from others. In this garden of pain and pleasure, we find our way.

Thrill of Risk

Risk is fun, dangerous, and a trigger for alertness. It may raise your testosterone and motivation. It gets you up and into action, but only some are into risk. Most or many shy away from it, but there is no gain without risk. So many people who like risk realize it's about managing risk. It's also a challenge for anyone. The challenge is to make a field, domain, or area of chaos, something you don't know, and then mine it for desired outcomes. What does this mean? When you find a risk you are attracted to, you look at it and figure out how to get through it, then take action, make mistakes, feel it, and mine it for what you love. I did it to see if I could do it. I did it because I wanted the experience. I take on challenges. Risk is fun, exciting, and motivating until someone gets hurt.

Risk? What Risk?

We take them all day long. Risk is offset by caution, preparation, and alertness. When we see danger, our senses go on high alert. We notice what is likely to injure or kill us, but if we have no experience, we don't know what to look out for. When we start something new, we approach it more cautiously. New places, people, and events can challenge us and keep our senses on high alert. It's stressful to start a new job, do something you've never done, or squeeze too much work in a short time. We live and die at risk. We love it and avoid it at the same time. With some effort, you can guess your risk and adapt accordingly.

Is riding a bicycle in New York City (NYC) safe?

So, I'm on a bicycle in NYC. It's raining and snowing, and the wind is blowing. I raise my hand to block the snow so I can see. I have my child riding between my arms. It's a bit cold. I know my risk is high, but I'm OK with it. My daughter is used to it. We've been doing it for six years. She doesn't complain. We are in our tolerance of risk. When we started bicycling, we didn't go out in the snow. We took short rides in pleasant weather. Eventually, we built up our risk tolerance. When we try something new, we work to figure out how difficult it will be to accomplish our goal. If we have experience, we have some idea of the risk involved. If it's something new, there's a risk that we have yet to encounter. Others have, and they've been through it; there's little risk for them because they are used to living and working through the risks they have chosen. After a while, we develop skills and forget we never knew how to do it. We move toward risk and danger to discover what the illusion will bring us. The illusion is that we will achieve the benefits or some unknown that we can't stop thinking about.

Risk Assessment According to Geography

Terry is a real estate investor. She is looking to buy a building but wonders about the area. From research, she finds out that the neighborhood could be better. There's high crime, bad schools, and vacant buildings. She compares this to another area with better schools, less crime, fewer empty buildings, and people with higher incomes. She reaches the risk of moving to that geographic area to others. She looks at the evidence and develops conclusions. With higher risk comes higher gain. Young and full of ambition, she moves toward the high-risk area and focuses on managing risk.

Geography of Danger

If you live in a small town, walk to work, and walk to most places, your risk of an accident can be pretty low. If you are a young man between 12 and 28 and live in a high-crime area, your chances of being a victim of a crime are higher. Avoiding dangerous people in dangerous areas is one line of defense. Selling drugs, breaking into buildings, and other criminal activity is hazardous and will increase your chances of injury and death. Drinking alcohol and driving compromises your safety and the safety of other people. If you live a life of danger, you either decide to quit or get closer to injury or death from unfortunate circumstances.

Risk Assessment Based on Time of Day

People use the light of day or dark of night to their advantage. A farmer plows in the day so she can see how to align her tractor. With modern machinery, the tractor is controlled via satellite to minimize fuel use and maximize efficiency. On sweltering days, the farmer may plow at night if she has satellite technology to guide the tractor. It's cooler at night, so the tractor may run more efficiently and break down less frequently. Another example comes from transport. I have errands to do on my bicycle. Using the internet, I discovered that the highest probability of an accident occurs an hour before and after sunrise and sunset. After work, people are eager to get home, perhaps tired from work and annoyed by other drivers. So, when I have the option, I avoid using the transport system when the probability of an accident is highest. Because I know when roads have the most dangerous drivers, I do my errands at other times.

Risk Assessment Based on Occupation

With economic changes, people lose jobs and change occupations. As they look for jobs, they assess how dangerous a job is. Some take advantage and find a job with less physical risk. All jobs have some risk, but how much? And what kind of risk? Sitting at a desk all day may seem easy to a construction worker, but that has risks, too. Office workers get carpal tunnel injuries, may have back problems, and suffer from indoor air pollution or eye-related stress from staring at a computer all day. A construction worker faces other dangers, including falling off scaffolds and ladders, tripping over tools and materials, injuries from using power tools, and exposure to toxic air, water, and materials. Most jobs have some level of risk. By researching, talking to industry employees, and learning the safety rules, it's possible to determine the level of risk of an occupation. If you have a choice, choose a job you can do safely.

Work Danger

Avoiding dangerous work should be a priority. Some enjoy the challenge and do it anyway. If you like dangerous work, you must be extra cautious to prevent much pain, suffering, and loss of income. Your supervisor should alert you about any dangers at work. If not, you must ensure you aren't injured on the job. You could also call a building inspector or the Occupational Safety and Health Administration (OSHA). They will come and inspect and may shut the job down. You may lose your job if the job is shut down. If it is shut down, it's better to lose your job than your life or have a bad accident. Another option is to list activities that seem dangerous to you. Ask your coworkers or supervisor how you can work safely. Ask if other workers have been injured doing your work. If so, make sure you know how to avoid those dangers. Do your research. It's your life; once you're injured, you may not be able to live the way you did before.

Danger for Manual and Skilled Workers

Many jobs that require physical labor are dangerous. If you are not alert, your chances of getting hurt or killed are much higher. Even workers with a pristine safety record must stay vigilant. Rushing through a job increases your risk. Long hours without sleep make a dangerous situation worse. Pushing hard and fast often generates low-quality work and injuries. Learning the safe way to work is essential and the fastest way to get work done. Proper training is crucial but often rare. It's your life and your body; learn how to work safely. It's a skill you can use for the rest of your life and teach others. If it doesn't look or feel safe, do something about it. Please write it down and talk to your fellow workers and supervisor. Be appropriate; the law may protect people who refuse to do unsafe work, but you must survive or at least get to the next step.

Job-related threats to your health.

Many jobs can destroy your health. Farmers, doctors, hospital workers, construction workers, and factory workers labor in dangerous conditions that are tough on the body and may ruin your health and well-being. For those who gravitate to the inchoate, for people who experiment and try risky procedures, injuries and accidents are more likely. Dangerous jobs require careful study and training to avoid accidents and injuries. Those with experience avoid difficult work conditions by thinking through the process, using the right tools and safety equipment, and following their gut instincts to prevent precarious procedures. If your body moves away from something and your mind triggers an avoidance response, it's time to take a step back and think about your actions. Break down goals into small steps. Identify the most risky procedures and find ways to make them safer. Clamps are like another set of hands. Jigs can hold things in place or provide a fence from danger. Before and during your day, remind yourself that your goal is to work safely, avoid danger, and work in ways that preserve the health and integrity of your body and mind.

Risk Assessment Based on Doctors Who Over-Prescribe Opiates

When people are hospitalized in pain, a doctor may prescribe opiates. If you have a weakness for getting addicted to alcohol, drugs, or opiates, you should be very careful. If you have family members, aunts, uncles, parents, grandparents, or ancestors with a history of drug abuse problems, you may have a genetic weakness for getting addicted to drugs. In recent years, many people have gotten addicted to opiates and have died after overdosing. If doctors make money prescribing the drugs, they may refill prescriptions while overlooking the patient's addiction. Some people get addicted to opioids, empty their bank accounts paying for the drugs, and wind up broke. With no money but still addicted, they turn to street drugs. If you don't have much experience, you may overdose or get AIDS or Hepatitis or related problems. One way to avoid going to a hospital is to steer clear of addictive drugs, including the ones prescribed by a doctor.

Patient Risk in the Medical System

Many want to avoid the medical system. It's littered with risk. Some medical procedures are invasive and have serious consequences. You could lose your life or suffer from complications. In the hospital, people are exposed to antibiotic-resistant bacteria and viruses that are not killed by drugs. Once infected, these diseases can be challenging to treat. Although hospitals use various methods to prevent medical mistakes, preventable medical errors kill nearly 100,000 people per year. Many actions must be done to make a procedure work correctly, so the probability of something going wrong can be high. Only if everyone does their job correctly will the procedure work. One way to minimize this risk is to bring a family member, friend, or advocate with you to the hospital. They can help you stand up and stop the medical system from pushing you into a procedure you don't want. When you are in pain, emotionally distraught, and facing an uncertain future, it's challenging to make decisions. Getting help from someone you trust is crucial. Perhaps if you focus on staying out of the hospital when you are in the hospital, you can avoid it in the future.

What are my Health Risks?

Health risks are activities you do that generate negative consequences for your health. I ride a bicycle in New York City. This is dangerous. Without extraordinary effort throughout a lifetime, I will likely be in an accident. I've been hit over five times by people opening their car doors and pushing me into other vehicles or on the street. Three times I hit the pavement after my front wheel ran into potholes, flipping me over the handlebars and into the pavement. I've walked away from all these accidents with minor scrapes and bruises. My family has a history of cancer and heart disease. My uncles and aunts who got these illnesses had habits which may or may not have influenced what happened. I do construction work. All day long, I'm exposed to different kinds of risk. I could drop something on my foot. I could fall off the ladder or scaffold. I could cut my finger with a tool. I can minimize my risk by paying attention and following safety procedures. What are the risks you face during the day? How can you minimize them?

Transport Risk

If you move, you risk injury. People love to move. A bicycle seems close to flying. Driving a car seems effortless but can easily result in tragedy. Car accidents kill 40,000 people per year and seriously injure many more. These are hazardous machines. Proper training and practice can improve your driving skills. Allowing extra time to make the trip is an excellent investment of your time. You can enjoy the ride and have time to enjoy the destination. If you are early, you could walk around the block and get to know the area. Using transit, bicycling, and walking have risks. People who walk and bicycle are closer to the source of pollution. Pedestrians, bicyclers, and transit users are constantly enveloped in toxic smoke. They don't have steel and glass in between them like a car. When you are exposed to weather, you feel the effects. The pain motivates people to take action. A vehicle can easily hit you regardless of your actions. You can reduce transport risk by assessing your risks and making goals and solutions.

Develop Good Habits

Beginning something new is a challenge. Motivation is key. When your mind and body are in good shape, your motivation is active, alive, and ready to go. Getting to that point may not be easy or likely. Many need more power to start something new. If your energy is low and you don't exercise or eat well, your body may not be ready for action. Good habits start one at a time. Step by step, keep going. Eventually, you will see the payoff.

Mortality Statistics

Probability, a statistical measure of the chance of an accident, gives us clues about how dangerous different activities are. When is a car accident most likely? At what time of day? What is the age and gender of a driver? If you know these statistics, will you avoid driving at night or become more alert when you see a young man behind the wheel? These statistics give us an idea of what is happening in our society. When more people die from poisoning than vehicle accidents, what is that telling us? Behind the scenes are significant trends that lead people to death. The society produces victims. Mortality statistics are fascinating and can help preserve your health by learning to avoid the most likely causes of death.

Statistic

The Centers for Disease Control and Prevention compiles statistics on the leading causes of death in the United States. Over time, it's possible to see trends. In 2016, the rate of opiate overdoses was significantly higher than the year before.

Number of deaths for leading causes of death:

- Heart disease: 614,348
- Cancer: 591,699
- Chronic lower respiratory diseases: 147,101
- Accidents (unintentional injuries): 136,053
- Stroke (cerebrovascular diseases): 133,103
- Alzheimer's disease: 93,541
- Diabetes: 76,488
- Influenza and Pneumonia: 55,227
- Nephritis, nephrotic syndrome and nephrosis: 48,146
- Intentional self-harm (suicide): 42,773

Death classified by mechanism of injury was highest from poisoning (26%), then transport accidents (16.9%), firearms (16.9%), and falls (16.5%). 80% of deaths by poisoning were not intentional. Death caused by non-intentional causes increased by over 7%. These numbers show how other people die and provide clues on what to avoid.

When to increase risk

Are you dissatisfied with your life? Do you want something more but need to know what it is or how to get there? Are you bored? Do you get jealous when you see other people doing something you wish you could do? Of course, step one is diet, exercise, stress management, and cultivating your mindset. Now, it's likely that you may want to charge into the good part right away. That would be to write about the best options to pursue. That's the big exciting part. What is going to be my next big challenge or next big adventure? Increasing your risk may require committing to something big; I will write one book per year. I will stop my job, make money, and have enough time to be the artist I've always wanted to be.

People take risks in order to gain something. At the same time, they estimate the danger and whether or not they will avoid going to the hospital. Mostly, people get it right, but the hospitals are full of people who didn't prevent injury. Often, with risk comes a danger. People take risks and negotiate through danger every day without injuring or killing themselves. Others underestimate the threat, get injured, and wind up in the hospital. With careful attention, embracing enough danger to keep alert is possible, but not enough to put you in the hospital.

CHAPTER 3
STRATEGIES TO MINIMIZE RISK

Risk is Unique to Your Ambitions

I risk; therefore, I am. Without risk, there is no change; without change, there is no improvement. Risk is exciting. I throw the dice. I know what I have to lose. I'm gambling with my life. Do I want to climb a steep wall of rocks without a safety harness? Do I ride a bike without a helmet or regard for traffic signals, bike lanes, and the safety of pedestrians? Most people who have suffered from risking too much realize the value of minimizing risk. Others who want to live 150 years have another strategy. If you wish to have a good time for a little while and let things happen as they will, that's another risk. Your risk depends on what you like to do and how you want to do it. If we think about risk, set goals, and make an effort, we can minimize danger.

Goals to Minimize Risk

If you make goals, you can direct action to meet your goals. Setting goals to reduce risk is possible, but first, I must know what risks I take. Most people have dangers at home, work, school, and transit. My safety risks at home can be reduced by checking smoke alarms, ensuring the stove is turned off when I leave home, and taking care while using the bathtub or shower. I can make a checklist and memorize it. As a first step, I can do this for home, work, school, and transit. If you learn to identify and minimize risk, you can apply similar methods to different activities. Risk is unique to the individual. My risks are different from many and similar to a few. Grow your list of risk goals, and you may become more confident about living safely.

Examples of Goals to Minimize Risk Time and Goal

By the end of the day today, I will list risky activities I face at home, at work, and when transporting.

In one week, I will finish my risk list and make a list of ways to reduce my risk. I will put this in a measurable format.

After one year, I will stop doing my riskiest activities, including not using safety glasses at work.

I will learn one new safety procedure each month until it becomes a habit.

The Carrot and Stick

With a goal in mind, we can move toward the goal. I want to wear a helmet every time I ride a bicycle, but why don't I wear one every time? Sometimes, we must look at what prevents us from realizing our goal. I want my hair to look good, but if I wear a helmet, it destroys my hair. I could change my hairstyle, wear a hat, or adjust my hair after I take my helmet off. If I practice a few times, I may generate a solution. So, we must remove impediments to our goal before achieving it. Next, we can remember what will happen if I don't reach my goal. Without a helmet, I could be injured or killed. Thinking of that can get me to put my helmet on real quick. Another reason could be that I want to see my friends or family when I get home. If I'm injured or dead, that won't happen. So, we want to remember what to avoid and why we want to reach our goal. This is a carrot-and-stick approach. When you think of your unique and personal reasons to do something, you are likelier to do it. One way to reach our safety and prevention goals is to use the carrot and stick method.

Strategies to Minimize Risk

List the main dangers in your life and ways to minimize the risk.

Set limits to your dangerous activities before you start.

Identify the most significant risks and ways to avoid those dangers.

So, what are some ways to minimize risk?

Live in a low-risk area in a low-risk country.

List and minimize high-risk activities at home, school, work, and when traveling.

Build your physical and mental performance.

Talk to fellow workers and bosses about minimizing risk and preventing accidents.

Grow a prevention or care team to minimize risk and prevent accidents.

Cultivate communities of care.

Avoid Risk

Some people avoid danger, and other people avoid risk. Risk implies a strategy to gain something. I'm risking jumping over the river to access the other side. The risk is that I will fall into the river, be injured, and drown. I could live my life to avoid risk. Taking it to the extreme would lead to death. I'm afraid of drinking water because I may be poisoned or I could choke on the water. All activity has risk. Fear of danger keeps us alive. We take risks all the time. After we are used to working safely, our risk goes down. We learn to avoid danger, have fun, and get work done. Risk something to gain something. You risk your safety to gain something else. You risk feeling uncomfortable to achieve something new in your life.

Accidents happen when people are tired, pushed to the limits, or working too fast. Schedule your most dangerous work when you're alert, without distractions, and have enough time, tools, equipment, and help. When you must push fast, make a safety checklist to help you avoid an accident. If I fail and there are few consequences, I fail quickly and try many things. The point is to be able to repeat how to do things the right way. If failure generates significant consequences, make a checklist to follow and proceed cautiously. The more risk, the more cautious you should be.

Goal Tactic

Avoid risky times Avoid driving during rush hour.

Avoid risky work Learn better safety practices or change jobs.

Avoid risky people Avoid drug addicts and careless people.

Avoid risky activities Avoid riding a bicycle at night when it's raining before and after sunrise and sunset.

Reduce Risk

Risk is the chance of an accident. I reduce my chance of an accident by keeping my brakes in good condition. I reduce the chances of an accident by eating well, exercising, and cultivating a proper mindset. I minimize the risk by going slower and approaching dangerous activities with more caution. I help others around me live safer so that they may do the same and my family and friends have less chance of being in an accident. An ounce of prevention is worth a pound of cure. It's much easier to prevent an accident than repair damage after an accident. If one of my friends or family is injured or ill, I may be available to help them get through it. I want to be on their care team, so they may want to be on mine. I want to be on their Care Team because it's very satisfying to help someone in need. I want to be on their Care Team to ensure they get the best care possible. If we look out for each other, a little effort can add up to a lot. This can make our world safer and more pleasant.

3 Foot Rule

Tools, materials, equipment, and workers occupy paths and scaffolds on a construction site. It's very active and dangerous, so workers must abide by the safety rules. One rule is the 3 Foot Rule. All paths, especially to exits, must be 3 feet wide. No tools, materials, equipment, hoses, or electrical cords can block the path. If you have experience on a construction site, you might say it's impossible. So, remember the three-foot rule in your house, on the street, or the job, and you'll make it safer. Keep all paths, especially egress, clear of clothes, junk, and garbage.

Egress

Firemen and women know about egress. So do architects and construction professionals. Egress is a path to an exit, usually a fire exit. Egress must be clear to allow safe and quick passage in an emergency. Some people wonder why public halls must be clear. After all, why can't we store a few things for a little while? What's wrong with that? If one person can do it, everyone can. That would lead to much stuff in the hallway and people competing for public space. You don't store your boat in a public park, right? Also, building and fire codes require egress to make it safe for occupants and emergency workers.

People need a clear path when carrying boxes, bags, and furniture. This makes it safer. Firemen and women, ambulance drivers, and emergency workers must be able to bring equipment and people in and out of the building quickly. Stuff in the hall can make this impossible and mean that an injured person dies or suffers more damage when they don't get to the emergency room fast enough. If you keep a clear path to exit an apartment or building, you can reduce the risk of an accident for your friends, family, or anyone else.

Reduce transport risk

For many people, an accident on the highways, streets, or stairs is their most considerable safety risk. Reducing transport risk is relatively easy but requires ongoing attention. If you get sleepy after lunch, it's best to drive after a nap, in the morning, or later in the day after a nap. Avoid rush hours, typically between 7 and 10 am and 4-7 pm late afternoon. If you can, take transit or carpool and let someone else drive. Transit, which uses professional drivers who drive the same route repeatedly, is safer and cheaper than driving, and you can read or sleep in transit. Walking and riding a bicycle may be another option. In some cities, bike lanes make cycling safer than it used to be. Usually, riding a bicycle is more dangerous than other methods. I've done it for 40 years without an accident that required medical attention; however, I may be the exception. If you ride a bicycle, follow the rules, stay in the bike lane, and always wear a helmet.

Reduce Work Risk

Even office jobs have risks. If you're a farmer, construction worker, or dancer, you might wonder if that's the case. Sitting on a chair all day, typing for four hours straight, or staring at a computer all day is not suitable for anyone. If you don't move, you don't burn calories, and if you put on weight, you increase your chances of getting cancer, heart disease, and diabetes. All jobs have health risks. Don't assume there are none. Find out what they are and take action to minimize risk. Ask your fellow workers or supervisor if they know anyone who was ever injured on the job. Find out what happened and if something will be done to prevent the same thing from happening. Just because you're healthy now and have never had an accident doesn't mean that it will continue. Research the health risks of your occupation. Find out what the riskiest procedures are and how to do them safely. Get the right equipment or training. Remind yourself before you go to work to avoid danger while maximizing safety for yourself and the people around you.

Reduce Play Risk

Why pay attention to safety when you're having fun? That's no fun —unfortunately, that's when accidents happen, when you aren't paying attention. You lose yourself in play and push the limits. As you do, you go too far, and that's when it happens. I was having a blast dancing. I felt great and noticed people seeing me having a blast. I was going in a circle on one leg, and with the other leg rocking back and forth, my leg slipped out of the socket. Two months later, I'm just about back to where I was before the accident happened. If I would have backed off just a little bit, I would have had more pleasure over the long run. Bliss has its price, and if you can learn to enjoy a bit of restraint with yourself and others, you can avoid a catastrophe. So, if it's you or someone close to you, enjoy a bit of attention to safety when you are having fun. It's a lot more pleasure than taking someone to the hospital when they are supposed to have fun.

Reduce Vacation Risk

Vacations on the beach, hiking, climbing rocks, and having fun; vacations are places to let your guard down and relax. Yes, I can do that, but there's a risk. If I'm hiking in the woods, do I want to stop and try to make it back on one leg because I tripped and sprained my ankle? I want to have fun, be wild, and know my safety limits. It's important to stop before the breaking point. Some of us learned the hard way; others learned from others and were smart enough to hold back enough to have some fun but not too much. Too much fun is when someone is injured and has to go to the hospital. At home, work, or vacation, we can strike a balance and take a risk, but not too much.

CHAPTER 4
BUILDING PERFORMANCE

Now and Forever
Your body either performs or doesn't. Of course, there are many grey areas. If you are alive, your body functions at some level. Maximizing your mental and physical skills is the goal of building performance. You're on the right track if you eat well, exercise, and minimize stress. If you make some goals, you will have a way to measure your progress and adjust your effort to meet your goals. You could do it formally and write it out with daily goals or do it by memory. Building performance is about generating the mindset to set and achieve goals to improve your mental and physical abilities. Motivation, herbs, and goals are fuels to make it happen. Building performance can reduce your chance of injury in an accident.

Building a Metaphor
Metaphors feed motivation. If you can build motivation, you can turn your body into the future, reach goals, and build confidence. Motivation, action, and experience build skill and confidence. My body moves like the flight of my favorite bird. I live a thousand and one dreams. I will use my energy to feed the future. Connect your metaphors to your goals. I want to exercise more every day. My energy is like Sisyphus pushing the giant bolder up the mountain; even though

it gets more arduous, nothing can stop me. Cultivate metaphors to share with others and fuel your body into action. Use this fuel to generate ways to stay ready for more action.

Effort and Practice

Chores can be an opportunity or a drag. It's a drag if you set your mind up to think it's a drag. It's an opportunity if you want to make someone happy or if you figured out how to enjoy this activity. I cleaned the kitchen and realized how good it looked when I was finished. I had some tea with friends, and we enjoyed an experience that would not have happened without me. Mindsets and interpretations shaped the experiences. Mindset requires effort and practice. The person you met who made you feel like you're the best person in the world didn't just pick the idea out of a hat. They are good at it and have done it many times. They orient their mind to find positive traits. You have done something to trigger their gracious interaction. If you can do some errands to help your community, consider it your chance to exercise and give people one more reason to keep you around.

Stay Motivated

Motivation is the key to making action happen and staying out of boredom, depression, and sitting on the couch. How can we feed motivation? Peak nutrition is crucial. This includes staying away from all processed foods while choosing peak-nutrition foods. Peak foods are loaded with vitamins, minerals, and complex compounds. The standards like garlic, ginger, bone broth, and whole fruits and vegetables are a good start. To add a tremendous amount of power and nutrition, take herbs. Ginseng-related herbs build power and motivation. Taking these can generate motivation by increasing your physical energy. Other herbs like alfalfa, oat straw, ginkgo, gout-kola, passion flower, damiana, and lemon balm feed the body and brain and open the mind to combat mediocre limitations. Mindset is crucial in this equation. Instead of moaning about carrying heavy things or doing chores, see it as an opportunity to increase your contribution to the household while building your muscle power and skills. People who can cook, clean, and fix things around the house are always more welcome than the couch potato who whines about doing the most minor chore.

Set Goals

Goals give you a target to move towards. With a goal, you can measure performance. Also, a goal can motivate you to keep going. Without a goal, it's easy to quit too soon. I feel tired when I hit 50 repetitions and wonder whether I can make it. When I know I want to go to 250, I keep pushing. I can do it since I've done it before. Performance is based on my ability to imagine doing what is impossible. Forget failure and keep pushing on. Imagine it will work. When you think they won't work, take a break or do something else; don't dwell on things not working. If things do fail, figure out a way to win. Yes, I didn't hit my goals, but I found out my limits and the next steps I have to take to reach my goals. I may have to reduce my goals to preserve motivation and safety. Think of defining your goal as presenting you, your desires, and your dreams to people.

Scheduling

This can be done in a formal or informal way, but when you make time to do something, it's more likely to happen. Many high-powered exercises can be done in a short amount of time. Twenty-five push-ups, 25 squats, or 150 bicycle pilates can be done in less than 30 minutes. The trick is to get started and keep doing it. One reward is to look in the mirror and observe your progress. Another is to imagine how good it feels to be strong. A muscular body may avoid injuries. You can do more sporting activities and take a brutal beating. Hard-worked muscles can feel good the next day.

Meditation

Your brain is most powerful when it's relaxed. The state of highest creativity is the time between being awake and asleep when you are at peak relaxation but not asleep. Your brain does well with oxygen. Give it more to give it a boost. Meditation brings peak performance to your mind. Meditation relaxes your mind, floods your brain with oxygen, and increases circulation. I've used meditation to calm down after being extremely agitated, both emotionally and intellectually. It's time to meditate when you are flustered, feel overwhelmed, or need to perform and figure out why you can't. Here's a straightforward method that takes practice to learn but pays off in a huge way when you need it.

How to Meditate

Imagine your lungs have a lower, middle, and upper section

Completely exhale

Inhale the bottom section of your lungs to the count of 5.

Inhale the middle section of your lungs to the count of 5-10.

Inhale the top section of your lungs from 10-15.

Hold your breathe to the count of 15

Exhale the top of your lungs from the count of 15 to 10

Exhale the middle of your lungs from the count of 10 to 5

Exhale the bottom of your lungs from the count of 5 to 0

Do it any number of times. Just do it.

This meditation floods your brain with oxygen and energy. It will help you relax when you are anxious or over-stressed or feel you are under an emotional or stressful attack. It takes to help you settle down so your brain can work. It will give you solutions when you are freaked out and don't know what to do.

The Reset Button: Meditation

Meditation is like a Reset Button for your Brain. It's a panacea to get back on track. As you focus on your breath, all the messages in your head driving you nuts fall away. The energy of the blood and oxygen feeding your brain break through the obnoxious, poisonous message that prevents you from realizing your goals. The more you focus on your breath, the more your focus returns. You understand what is important and can stand up for yourself. When you're off balance and feel like you are falling, it's there. It's there when you need someone and they can't or won't come. Make meditation your friend that never fails. Anytime you're waiting and want to boost your mind, it's there. Tap into the power of your lungs and discipline. Tap into your friend; meditation.

Benefits of Meditation

Feed your mind for peak performance.

Calm down after someone attacks you in a physical, emotional, or spiritual way.

Use it to collect your thoughts so you can make the right decisions.

It can be done anywhere, anytime, and requires no money.

It can help you get through difficult situations.

When to meditate

When you are agitated after someone attacks you.

When you need mental energy to get work done.

When you feel lost and need to get grounded.

When you are flustered and overwhelmed and want to get back on track.

When you have a few moments while waiting for someone or something.

Whenever you want a boost.

Practice and Let the Air Flow

You must learn and practice meditation. It's a skill. The more you do it, the easier it gets. Once you know and stop doing it, you will get rusty but should be able to pick up again. So, meditation is in your toolbox. It can maximize the performance of your brain. It can help you focus when other people or circumstances flood your mind with too much stress. Within five minutes, I've used this technique to go from highly agitated to a state of mind where I'm clear, focused, and figure out what to do. Learning to meditate pays off in significant ways. Once you know it, you can use it for the rest of your life. You don't need money, other people, or special tools. You can do it anywhere, anytime. Meditating can keep you out of the hospital and help you make decisions when stressed out. It's a way to add power to your brain. It is a way to feed oxygen and blood to the brain, minimize distraction, and be in a state of total relaxation.

How to Build Up Your Health

Making goals that become habits is a way to transform your life. Start slow and develop momentum. Find a way to grow pleasure into the routines you engage in. Take activities you like least or most significant weaknesses and find ways to make them pleasant. Choosing what you eat and how you exercise can become a way to gain traction in your life. Use that traction to go beyond your life and move into the person you want to be. I make goals and slowly move toward them. My friend takes an idea and develops it over 20-50 years. He adds occasionally and constantly makes little adjustments to grow something beyond. Take your life and make those little improvements that make a big difference. Take on massive projects that last 30-50 years or longer. Use them to give your life meaning and purpose. This can keep you strong, active, and motivated.

Here are some goals to build up your health:

Eat two servings of fresh food each meal.

Eat to have enough fuel to get to your next meal.

Eat to maximize the nutritional difference. Drink and use many herbs.

Begin making regular attempts to exercise.

Set goals to build the core abs with pilates, push-ups, and squats.

Learn to boost immunity and healing with greens and power herbs.

10% of Peak

Building up your body means increasing your physical and mental performance so that you are within 10% of your peak capacity when you need it. Get to know your limit so that you can approach your limit, but don't injure yourself. As you take risks and meet goals, you will gain confidence. Use your energy to move ahead. Do it in a smooth, graceful way that empowers people along the way. Knowing your limits helps you say no to things that may push you over the edge and wind up in the hospital.

Simple Steps

Make simple steps to improve your health. Every morning, I will do one exercise that takes less than five minutes. I will do the same every afternoon, and in the evening, I will do another round.

In the morning, I will do my bicycle pilates.

In the afternoon, I will do push-ups.

In the evening, I will do squats.

Simple Steps Impossible Goals

Impossible goals are fascinating. Without chaos and disorder, you have nothing to work with. Once you find the impossible, you have something. It's not some absolute requirement; it's something to play with, to ponder as you frolic through your day. A challenging goal keeps you motivated to continue but can also wear you down and make you get depressed. Learn when to take a break and let it go for a while. This can help a lot, but you must start again, which can take significant effort. Write your goals down and look at them at night and in the morning. Concentrate your energy and make-do lists to make action happen to keep you healthy and ready for action.

Focus on the Core Area to Prevent Big Problems

Your back and stomach muscles connect your legs and hips and hold your body together. If you do manual labor that requires lifting, you will have fewer problems if you strengthen your core muscles. Your chances of getting a back injury decrease as you learn to lift correctly and develop good posture. With confidence that your core is strong, you won't hesitate to do the heavy lifting or other tasks requiring a solid back. I do bicycle pilates. I saw them in a television commercial. Slowly, I learned how to do them. Now, I do them once every day or two. They take about 5 minutes. I rarely have a back problem or back pain. I can lift heavy things and do serious work without a problem. My abs look OK, which I enjoy. It takes effort to develop good habits, but it pays off. When your core is strong, you gain confidence. Strengthen your core by doing bicycle pilates, push-ups, and squats. These will make you strong without going to a gym or taking special pills.

Medical Journal

Keeping a medical history can help you organize your health records in a coherent way. It will help you to identify what works quickly and doesn't work to help you heal through injury and illness. You could also use it to help you organize your Care Team. The journal could have a written component and a spreadsheet. One is a diary or written explanation of what happened when you got sick and how you overcame it. The other is a database with dates, times, names of doctors and helpful people, what works and doesn't work, what websites to use, and other things that help you move through injury and illness. One section could focus on your goals and how well you met them. Did I accomplish the goals on time? Were the results the quality that I wanted? Keeping a medical journal and spreadsheet can help you focus and take control of your medical health.

Benefits of a Medical Journal

Use it to diagnose your illness or injury.

You can track what works and doesn't work.

Track your family's medical history and ways to counter genetic weakness.

Strategically make goals to counter your genetic weakness.

Use it to track your goals to eat well, exercise, control stress, and develop mindset goals.

Keep a record of your doctor, hospital, and dental visits.

Rate the performance of medical professionals and note what they do well and not do well.

Help track your medical contacts.

It helps you see the bigger picture and make little adjustments to make significant changes.

Use it as a hobby tool, play around and enjoy it, and make it your information treasure.

When you get good at it, help other people do it.

Simple Toolbox for Building Performance

Diet

Exercise

Stress Reduction and Meditation

Develop and Achieve Mindset Goals

Diet

This is a straightforward diet. Start with 2-3 servings of fresh, uncooked fruits and vegetables for each meal. Center your meals around fresh foods. Try to eat 1-2 salads each time. The second idea is to eat the minimum required for your next meal. Remember that the less you eat, the more energy you will have later. Overeating turns me into a beached whale. Don't stare at the food. Look at it, go for fresh food, and eat as slowly as possible. Aim for quality, nutrition, and high-energy food. Stay away from all processed food. Eat whole foods as much as possible.

Exercise

Make goals to build up your core. The core is your muscles holding your back, legs, arms, and head together. Squats, bicycle pilates, and push-ups are three essential exercises you can do without a gym, without money, and without much time to make your core super strong. Aerobic exercise is also crucial. At least 2-3 times per week, you should exercise your heart for 20 minutes at 2/3 of its capacity.

Stair climbing works if your building has a good set of stairs. Running, jogging, and playing sports also work. Keep in mind that to get strong requires serious effort. Develop your myths and mindsets to power yourself ahead. Think of the big, strong stars that inspire you. Just make goals and keep at it. Go slow and develop traction and momentum. This pays off over and over, day after day, without failure. One goal is to do any exercise until the pain is not fun, then take a break and keep going. If each exercise is not overly painful and pleasant, building the strength of your body may come quickly.

Stress Reduction and Mindset Goals

Some things matter, and some things don't. When I tried to find out what mattered, I narrowed it down to one thing: the health of my family and friends. I don't need to get excited about all the other stuff; it may be different for you. I can't and don't want to control people or things. I'm one person on this planet in this universe. I will come and go and mostly will be forgotten. I'm here and now. To keep my stress OK, I keep these things in mind. Let go of things that drive you nuts, be agile in your interpretive regimes, and use compassion and empathy to dissolve your anger. Do the best you can and be happy with that. Do things for others to keep them happy; it's easier than hearing them whine and complain. Develop your mindset goals by using them as a path to realize your desires and dreams. Integrate your mindset goals into the groups of people you want to be with. Use your mindset goals to be the change you want to see, to be the person you want to be and develop a healthy, happy life with the people around you.

Circulation in Your Brain

Exercise, herbs, and meditation can increase blood circulation to the brain. Why is circulation so important? Your brain is made up of many small nerves and blood vessels. The blood vessels feed the nerves. When you exercise, you maximize the energy flowing through your blood to your nerves. Keeping your blood vessels in good shape is essential. One herb, gout-kola, is good for blood vessels and capillaries. It keeps them strong and functioning well. Cayenne is also good for circulation. I've made a mix of olive oil, garlic, salt, rosemary, and cayenne. I dip bread in it and feel a tingling in my brain for a minute.

It's nearly similar to scratching with your fingernails on the scalp of your head. It feels good and helps the blood flow to your brain.

Maximizing Mental Performance

Your mind is a muscle. To do well, it requires the right inputs. Garbage in, garbage comes. Diet, exercise, and stress control significantly impact your mind. Herbs like gingko, gotu-kola, and rosemary are suitable for your brain. These have unique compounds that other plants and medicines don't have that help your brain function. Some herbs remove toxins that reduce your mental performance. Exercise pumps blood to your body. With peak oxygen levels from exercise, your mind will operate higher. Stress control includes meditation. Meditating can radically improve your ability to think and process emotional energy that may block you from realizing your goals. Meditation relaxes your brain while maximizing the blood and oxygen in your brain. The mind is most creative in a state of relaxation. The time between when you are awake and fall asleep is a period of peak performance for your mind. At times, you become aware of it. This happens moments before you jump out of bed after realizing a great idea.

CHAPTER 5
AWARENESS TO AVOID INJURY

wareness meets action

Awareness is the crown jewel of action that you can use to avoid a hospital visit. After your body and mind exercises, you can fine-tune awareness, but what is awareness? Awareness is the alertness of the mind. It's the ability to think quickly and notice what is at hand, in front of you and all around. It's the ability to interpret multiple perspectives simultaneously to respond appropriately. Ideally, you can generate awareness that prevents accidents without cramping spontaneous fun. When fully aware, we can scan our environment, note what is most important, and choose appropriate actions that keep us on track.

Awareness is Multiple

Awareness is a skill. Look at an experience and find multiple interpretations. Each interpretation opens or closes options. When you come upon something, you look at it from a particular perspective. You may or may not be aware of it. You are drawn to it. It draws me in: that red color, the method of delivery, the quality of the sound, or the intent that made something happen. You are looking for something and don't know what it is. You are looking for something and need to learn how to look for it. You take steps in a direction. If you keep your interpretations open, you have more options. You have yet to learn; you have to do more research and find out what is going on. If you approach a phenomenon as multiple, you have more options. Something is blocking awareness. Take a few steps back and see another angle. Go for a walk and let it go for a while. Meditate or write about it. Sometimes, those options lead us away from the hospital into another method or goal. By opening up the experience and seeing multiple, we gain more options that prevent a hospital visit.

Change and Growth "Fail, fail better" Justin Smith.

Everyone makes mistakes. What do we do with those "mistakes?" Some people write them down and throw them in the garbage. Others write them down, talk about it, and make a plan of action to avoid that behavior. Mistakes can be difficult to talk about. If we state and bring out our mistakes, we may be more likely to do something about it. I pay attention, and now I'm aware that I did something to hurt someone else or something that caused problems or pain for someone or something. By talking, writing, and making plans of action, you can avoid making your mistakes over and over. Conditions breed mistakes. You explode when you are under pressure to leave the house and can't find your keys. On Friday nights, when we are hanging out, we like to have a couple of drinks, but it gets late, and eventually, you are too tired and drunk, so you pass out on the couch. Ultimately, you find ways to avoid the wrong behavior or suffer the consequences. You learn to make decisions. You begin to say no. You realize that you must do something else instead of your bad behavior. To grow, we have to change. We grow out of one thing and into another. We move away from risky behavior to less risky behavior. If we can fail better, it's enough to stay safe.

Conditions for Awareness

One key to prevention is keeping your mind active, alive, and alert. A healthy mind grows in the health of your body, family, and community. A person reflects the family, school, and community that cultivates the conditions for a person to grow, fail, and keep going. If you learn to surround yourself with people who support your growth and development, you are more likely to realize your highest potential without injury.

Foundation of Awareness

The body is a foundation for the energy of the brain. The brain requires fresh blood and oxygen to do well. Maximizing the body's power to produce energy requires food, exercise, and a mindset. Nothing happens without effort. Often, the more effort you put in, the more you get out. Keeping aware requires constant effort. If you bicycle in New York City, you either pay attention or end up in an accident. Often, the danger makes people more alert, which is why some people seek danger. They like to maximize alertness with danger and, in the moments of danger, focus intently on what is going on. Peak alertness can minimize danger, maximize safety, and prevent accidents.

Choosing Critical Variables

Developing awareness is like seeing 360 degrees at all times. Scanning and choosing crucial variables is a skill people develop. This applies to art, engineering, putting on makeup, and skilled trades like carpentry, welding, and plumbing. First, you look for the critical elements that make the difference for your goal. I need to move that pipe over a half inch to make it level; what is in the way? I want to turn my bicycle through traffic in the safest way possible; what route should I take to maximize safety for me, my child, pedestrians, and vehicles? The more I can stay out of the way, the better. Riding a bicycle in heavy traffic requires confidence. Eventually, you will be able to choose one route among many. The route you choose should maximize safety and efficiency.

Research

It's your life; put more in and get more out. Staying out of the hospital requires effort and perseverance. One step ahead of the rest of the population will help you prepare for the worst and hope for the best. What was common knowledge before may not be so common now? Before the internet, you couldn't just type a few words into a search engine and expect results. For some groups, life expectancy is going down; for others, it's increasing. When you know how people are dying, you can take steps to avoid it. Changing your diet, exercising, and reducing stress are common areas for improvement. If you know that people of your gender, age, and occupation are dying more frequently than years ago from job-related injuries, you could research how to work safer and adopt safer habits.

Expectations

If you expect to die in a couple of years, how would you live? If you wish to live another 50 years, how would you live? How would you change your life if you knew you must live to be 150? What if something happened, and you knew you could live another 500 years? How would you live? Expectations change how people live now. Will my neighborhood be underwater in 20 years? This will influence what people do now. If you move out before the flood, you will probably get a better price for your property. If you are renting and a flood destroys large areas of the neighborhood, you may not want to live there. If you thought you had to live to be 150, perhaps you would change your safety procedures.

Medical Logs and Spreadsheets

Awareness is a deeper understanding of your body's health to heal better. Using a computer spreadsheet can help you make a plan to heal better. Keeping a log of what worked and didn't work can prevent confusion and help create an action plan. Depending on your situation, these could become quite complex. The organization makes a big difference. Start with basic information including date, description of illness or injury, healing plan, methods and herbs or medicine used, people consulted, doctors and hospitals. If you like to write, then write it out. Use a technique that works for you. Read and revise or add something to it. Look for patterns. Am I doing the same thing, and it's not working? Who helped me the most? Did I get more from researching than a doctor's visit? Look for what works and doesn't work. Take enough time to set this up, go slow, make sure it makes sense, and consider how to use and improve it. This is a valuable information bank. Use this information to fine-tune and enhance your awareness of your body and how it heals to stay healthy.

CHAPTER 6
GOALS AND HABITS

Goals are the significant steps that define your life. I want to write a book and travel around the world. Habits are little steps that lead to a goal. I need to write one chapter per week. I will work on that for 3 hours in the afternoon and write 1500 words daily. When a goal seems too complicated, break it down into small, manageable steps. If you get stumped, keep breaking down the goal until the steps are easy. Take your time with steps. The more you work through the whole process, the easier it gets. Remember, experience is the best teacher. Habits form as we work through an activity. We can use benchmarks to guide and improve our habits if we have benchmarks that lead to our goals. Using a spreadsheet or checklist can make it more thorough and systematic. Over time, we develop more skills and confidence. As you realize little goals, your confidence will grow. After you meet your larger goal, you will be inspired to take on another one. Goals guide action, and action generates skills, habits, and confidence. Let your goals and habits lead you to a better life where you are confident about caring for yourself and others. Use goals and habits to minimize your chances of winding up in the hospital.

Habits Become Goals

A goal has a result and a timeline. By April 1, 2017, I will do five push-ups per day. I will do one more each week until I'm up to 25. Each day or two, I will do 50 bicycle pilates. After learning the basics of an exercise, I no longer think about how to do it. It becomes a habit. Goals turn into habits. Once they are habits, they are done with less effort. I don't need to learn the fundamentals. Goals are achieved with motivation and power. Getting off the couch requires motivation. Eating well, exercising, and cultivating a proper mindset will feed motivation to help you realize your goals.

Goals can reduce the chances of going to the hospital. Here are some goals:

1. Do exercises 3-4 times per week

I will do 10-25 squats 3-4 times per week, which takes less than 10 minutes each time.

I will work up to 25 push-ups 3-4 times per week; these take less than 10 minutes.

I will do stair climbing 3-4 times per week; this takes 20-25 minutes.

2. I will eat two servings of fresh food thrice daily.

3. I will list my risky activities and plan to reduce them. I will do this twice weekly, using 10-15 minutes.

4. I will practice meditation and mindset building three times per week, which could start with 10-15 minutes a day.

5. I will research questions I have three times per week for 20 minutes each time.

Goal Setting Skills

One function of a goal is to motivate me to take action. I can change how I think, write, and speak about goals. I want to use goals for motivation. How do I work to achieve my goal if distractions stop me? Here's one way. Break a goal into steps and estimate how much time to spend on each step. Let's say for 1 goal, you break it down into five steps, each taking an hour. Now, I know how to meet my day's goal. I took five steps that lasted one hour. I also like doing other things, like reading papers, posting on social media, finding a new recipe, or designing a garden plot. Here's a way to motivate yourself to achieve all your goals. If I finish my hourly goal before 60 minutes, I can use the other time to do the lower-priority items. I have to get my highest-priority work completed first. It's possible to design your goals to increase your motivation.

Goals in Format

A format for a goal is: I have a goal. It has a beginning, middle, and end. I focus on the goal in the morning and at night. I write the goal and paste it on the board, on the wall, or in my head. It's made of stone. I connect with my goal. I memorize it, meditate on it, look at it, speak about it, make art, and become intimate with my goal. I'm connected in a unique, authentic, and personal way. I make the goal me, and the goal makes me. I feel the power of the goal as it unleashes me into action. Goals guide action, give direction, and give my life a purpose. The format of the goals is a hint of the method. The method connects the beginning of the goal to the end of the goal. Procedures can be fluid and multiple. Look at someone who is good at what they are doing. Since they have worked through many problems, they know shortcuts and tricks to get through issues other people get stuck on. Those who are stuck stop moving. The format for a goal could be benchmarks. These are achievements that must be completed to reach your goal.

Habits

Habits are activities you have learned that you do repeatedly without pushing hard to get started. It's something you don't have to think about or plan or make a lot of effort to do. When I leave the apartment, I look for trash or recycling to take down the stairs. It's one of the contributions I make to my household. One goal is to maximize the little things I can do to help make my community work. If I can make delicious, nutritious dinners quickly, I can keep people happy and satisfied. I can take pleasure in seeing them enjoy the food I've made. My habits become a contribution. My contributions are another reason people want to keep me around. If I make a habit of being the first one to volunteer to get something done, I may generate some good karma. Good habits lead to better consequences. With my habits, I can make a community. A community of people who look after and help each other stay out of the hospital. In this book, habits lead to goals that help me stay healthy. Typically, this means diet, exercise, stress reduction, and cultivating a mindset.

Habits and Goals

If I'm going to change my habits, I've got to have a goal. This will direct what I'm doing and keep track of my progress or regress. I want to do 25 push-ups 4-6 times per week. I've got something to shoot for. It is best to write down the goal and post it on the wall, door, or my notebook. The point about a habit is not that I do 25 push-ups the first time. It's all about making something automatic. The first time you start, it's something new and different. It takes a while to finish the first attempts. Make enough time to get accustomed to the habit you are forming. Choose a time of day, place, and method. Just aim to be consistent and track your progress. Don't push it; try to make it comfortable and easy. You need to cultivate motivation. If you go too hard, you will suffer an injury, which might stop you from doing it again. As time passes and you learn better methods, you can improve your performance. Often, the most challenging thing to do is to start. It's to get off the couch and get moving.

Changing Habits Can Change Your Life

Habits form slowly. Eating is a habit. I eat for pleasure, or I eat for pleasure and nutrition, or I eat for nutrition first and pleasure later. I care less about how food tastes than how it will improve my mental and physical performance. So, how do I get started? Let's say I want to change my eating habits. I want more nutrition. This may work for some people, but it won't give you all the benefits. You may become open to eating more fruits and vegetables. The point is that you can easily change your health by eating more fresh food. One way is to create a goal to eat at least two servings of fruits and vegetables per meal.

What habit?

Eating is a habit, a necessary one. We all do it all day long. Eating two servings of fruits and vegetables per meal can make a huge difference. To get started, do it and keep doing it. In the morning, perhaps an apple, orange, banana, and whatever vegetables you have around. Mustard greens and eggs are great, and so are many other combinations. Put them in your mouth, chew, and swallow. It's that easy, but it could be challenging for many. Some people develop a friendship with a plant they love. They learn to grow, harvest, store, and eat it.

Meanwhile, a friend keeps giving comfort, health, and nutrition. Here, the habit is to make a friendship relationship with plants or animals or hobbies. These are different from your typical friends. Making friends becomes a habit. I use the method of making friends and apply it to plants, animals, hobbies, and people. I have a habit of making goals and habits. When I have nothing else to do, I'll start writing down, speaking about, and making goals and habits—first, the goal, then the habit.

Develop Healthy Hobbies

Hobbies can make habits that generate big dividends. Learning to grow and use herbs is an example. Start simply by finding an easy-to-grow plant and a place to plant it. Or find some peppermint tea and see how much pleasure you can get from drinking it. Putting a few minutes or more daily into it can yield significant results. It's also a way to fill your day with joyous activities, especially if you want to stop a bad habit or change the focus of your life. Growing and using herbs is an ongoing project that can satisfy your appetite for physical and mental challenges. Making soil and planting and harvesting herbs is pleasant work that can keep you active without risking too much injury or stressing your body too much. Researching how to grow and use herbs provides your brain with problems that motivate action. Developing healthy hobbies is a way to enhance your life and the lives of those around you. It's also a good answer when people ask what you are doing with your life. Using herbs to stay healthy and helping others do the same is a fun, healthy hobby.

Think Numbers

If you think in numbers, you can measure your performance. I want to write 500 words per day. I will swish this turmeric around my mouth up and down ten times, side to side ten times, and all around ten times, and let it in my mouth for 10 minutes. By putting numbers on it, you can measure progress or regress and adjust your goals as you monitor the results. Just make it a habit or hobby and experiment or play with it. Approach each new thing like an experimental tinker toy. This is another way to cultivate goals, habits, and awareness. Doing this makes it easier to communicate. I can tell someone an exact number of range of numbers. It's also another chance to play with math. By thinking in numbers, you can develop habits that help you think through goals that can keep you out of the hospital. Every day this week, I will wear my bicycle helmet when I ride my bicycle. I use my goals and habits to improve my life, gain power and control, and enhance and invigorate my life and those around me.

Staying Out of the Hospital with Goals and Habits

Use goals and habits to reduce your chances of going to the hospital. These can make your life more pleasant, active, and sustainable. Goals that focus on eating well, exercise, stress reduction, and cultivating mindset are an excellent place to start. Your performance and confidence will grow as you form goals and turn them into habits. You will learn new skills that enhance your life and those around you.

CHAPTER 7
GROWING A CARE TEAM

Organize a Care Team

If you learn how to organize a care team, you will have more security about your health and well-being. One of the most challenging things about being sick or injured is to ask for help. It will be easier if you have a mutually supportive relationship with someone. Here are a few ideas to get started. A care team has members who do what they can to help you. They may differ from what you want, but you must work with who you have because you may not get who you want the most. Who do you want on your care team? The best are people who you trust and people you have worked with in the past. If you have worked with someone as a volunteer or in a cooperative setting, you can understand what they need to perform well. If you've been working together, you can ask and give things when needed. The best is to lead by example. Offer help to people you are close to; eventually, they may reciprocate. Of course, it's essential to choose the people you help wisely. If they constantly complain after you help them, you may hand off the activities to another person. Sometimes, this is impossible, and then you must mine the experience for what it is and how you extract pleasure and satisfaction from it. Some people are complicated. You don't want to jeopardize your health and happiness.

Ideally, it's a large group of people caring for a small number of people. If you're good at organizing, that can be a significant benefit.

A care team helps you stay well, get better when you are not well, and use a hospital when needed. These are people you can trust. If you develop a relationship where you help someone first, they may help you later. Often, family and friends are an excellent place to start. Another option is to volunteer somewhere and connect with fellow workers. Invite them to a potluck and tell them to bring a friend. Tell them you want the focus of the potluck to be on making a care team. Teams work when there is a culture of help in the community. If you care for your community, they will take care of you. If they need you and you need them, it becomes a community of mutual support. If it's good for my community, it's probably good for me. As I get to know people in my community, I can trust others to decide for me. I support their choice, even if it makes me twitch a little. I'm not going to agree with everything my community does. However, I do expect them to consider my input and give me an answer as to why they chose something else. A community of care takes care of each other.

Why do I need help?

When you are sick or injured, your ability to care for yourself may be compromised. You may not be able to get food, go to work, or take care of others. Often, resourceful people will figure out how to do it on their own. However, that's not always possible. When you can't take care of yourself and have no family or friends to turn to, you may have to go to the hospital until you are well enough to take care of yourself. Social service agencies may help. Now, you must go out of your way to ask people for help. You must do this to everyone around you and hope for the best. This is a challenging position, so when you are healthy, you want to work on staying healthy and put some effort into making a care team.

Community Oriented Care

People can live more efficiently in numbers. Some people do OK alone or in a small group of 1 to 3 people. Others see the value of a larger group and move in that direction. Larger groups can be organized to meet the needs of the community. This allows people to specialize in one function, enjoy doing different functions, and take advantage of the specialized skills of various members. Many have no idea how to live with other people. The idea that they should cook for 10-20 people rather than for themselves is quite a stretch. These people may benefit by getting more education. For people who have never lived in a community, doing work jobs, going to meetings, and working for everyone, not just myself, may be difficult. Most co-ops have 10-20% who do a lot of the work and 20-60% who do just enough or just a little extra. The remaining 10-30% do the least they can and sometimes sabotage what is happening. Ideally, people see each other more for what they give than what others expect of them. In a community where people focus on the needs of many, caring for members may be more acceptable.

Family Oriented Care

A healthcare team can start with your family. Parents develop skills as they help their children grow through illness and injury. Keeping a cool head when your child is screaming in pain is not easy. Sometimes, you must make quick decisions with enormous consequences, so preparation is critical. Often, when a parent can't handle a screaming child, they turn to the Internet, call a nurse, and, if required, take their child to the hospital. If a grandparent or relative is available with skills, they may be consulted and may help out. This is one model of a care team. People without a family may have friends who take care of each other. Many families that need care have little power.

Parents may work two or three part-time jobs and have little time for anything else. They may be doing this and need help to keep up. Making alliances with neighbors to help each other out can work, but it has challenges. Some families have extended family living at home or close to home, which can help. Families bonded by blood and proximity can make a care team. Some members may not like or get along with each other. With effort, they may be able to make a care team, but this may require significant effort, especially if people need more money. People with money can hire people and tell them what to do. They don't have to work with the group and won't get the benefits of the group. The motivation and performance of a hired hand are much different from those of a group of people who are bonded by emotions, ideas, and experiences.

Make community

A community that openly shares resources like food, clothing, and shelter may help you get well. Mutual aid and self-help can buffer the trauma of a painful illness. Relationships require time and effort to establish and sustain themselves. They grow over time and need fuel to keep them active. Meeting regularly can form a structure to help a group continue. Parents can host a pizza night on Friday nights that allows elementary kids to bond and share stories of the week as they transition to the weekend. When communities form or let new members in, it's best to state what they expect from each other. If you say from the beginning that each person is expected to help out when someone gets sick, members can prepare to do their best before their efforts are required.

Ideal team

An ideal team works together smoothly and efficiently without intense conflicts that prevent people from working together. People with experience know how to negotiate through conflict. An organized group that defines work functions for each member is in an excellent position to organize assisted living functions. If the community is established and has members who aren't overburdened with other tasks, the community can absorb a sick person or two.

Online Support Groups

Most people with an illness are motivated to find a solution. This can be powerful. Finding other people who share your pain can provide positive support to boost your attitude. Seeing other people do what you want can inspire you to act. With Skype and FaceTime, you can connect in a more intimate way than just a phone conversation. Patients may also be able to demonstrate a procedure, show you special equipment, or show you different medicines that could help you heal faster. Online support groups are another way to connect with people with similar interests and may help you avoid traveling through hospital doors.

Organize A Care Team

Another approach may work. One can organize a care team by posting notices on the Internet. You must screen people carefully, be well organized, and offer something to get the team on the right track.

Craigslist and Meet-Up may be a place to start. Sometimes, people with similar illnesses and injuries bond well. This could be done in person or online. A great deal of support can be had over the phone or Internet. It's what you make it. When people are in need, they find solutions using what they have. By keeping this in mind, you can ignore those voices in your head that tell you it's impossible to organize a care team. It may work if you clearly state what you want and what you can give in return. You can barter hours or meals or a resource or skill that others don't have that you have too much of. Starting when people don't have health issues is a place to start. A potluck dinner at each person's house may get the ball rolling. It needs to be organized so people stay focused on the Care Team. If people commit to the idea, they may not even need to be there. Setting appointments, ordering food, and picking up medicine can be done without being there. They could offer to help or find someone to help when needed. Being open and flexible can make the process go smoother.

What does a Care Team do in a hospital?

Make sure the doctor knows what you want, and push to get it, even when the doctors move in another direction.

A care team is your eyes—ears, and brain when you are in too much pain to look out for yourself.

A care team observes and records what happens at the hospital.

A care team helps you make an informed decision and supports your decision.

Do List

Do lists prevent procrastination and distraction. You have a goal if you add a time period to each task. The goal is measurable, and you can gauge your performance to estimate how long it will take to do some future activity. If you keep an eye on the time, you may stop getting distracted and look at the news, weather, or other distractions. A do list must be coherent by consulting the larger goal and integrating the smaller goals into the larger goal. I'm getting my teeth fixed. I need to find a dentist, get a diagnosis, and get treated. I make the list and work through it. I've got to finish the first step to get to the second. I need to complete the first goals to get there. Do lists are little goals that lead to the big goal that leads to habits? Working through my lists can help me accomplish my goals, which can keep me out of the hospital.

Methods

Challenges require methods to realize a goal. Those with years of experience have a toolbox of methods to achieve what they are working on. They easily switch methods to achieve desired results. With flexibility, they can go beyond where they've been and do what needs to be done. As you set goals to realize a care team, be flexible and open to different methods. Inevitably, you will hit roadblocks that seem invincible. Write down what is stopping you from realizing your goal. Then, write questions about the roadblock. Now, try to answer them. Keep working through this process. If you do it 5-10 times, you may find a method worth doing. Then, do internet searches and see what happens. Are my methods and solutions similar to other people? If so, in what ways does it make a difference?

Care Teams Can Offer Comfort and Security

Setting up and using a Care Team is rare. You may be doing some of it and not realize it. Most families care for each other. They put together a unique version of a care team. If it works for them, great. If not, it may be an excellent time to try something else. Collective living is uncommon in most of the United States and may be a good start for a care team. Many are taught to hustle for money and assume everything else will fall into place. Caring for others is not an ordinary skill. Often, people who have suffered can empathize and be compassionate. They develop empathetic reflexes, and caring comes easily and naturally for them. Learning to care for people is a rewarding experience. If you want to feel deeper intimacy, this may be one option. People come alive in other ways when they go through hardship. A care team can empower you when you are sick and injured. They will help you get the food, herbs, medicine, and medical help to stay out of the hospital or get well fast when you must go there.

CHAPTER 8
INSURANCE

The United States has a private medical system with a public system to fill in the gaps. Usually, you see a doctor who checks for problems. If they see nothing, they let you go, and if they find something they can't deal with in their clinic, they refer you to a specialist. To see the doctor, you must meet the receptionist first. If you have insurance, you go to the next step, which is the nurse or a doctor. They may treat you in the emergency room if you don't have insurance. They are required by law to do so. They send you to a hospital with an emergency room. Here, you may or may not wait a long time. It depends on how injured you are and how busy the hospital is. The emergency room sees patients who need it the most and continues as doctors, nurses, and medical equipment become available. So, what's so complicated?

Private Health Insurance The Malaise of the Insurance Juggernaut

Private insurance provides a customer with healthcare insurance. You pay a premium, and they deliver according to the contract. The function of private health insurance is to make money. Their interests are separate from yours. They seek specific markets to specialize in. They target illnesses and injuries they can make money on. It's a fragmented, busted system that doesn't maximize beneficial relationships. To make money, they have to deny coverage and benefits. They shrink benefits, drop people when they get sick and refuse or delay payment to providers. Insurance companies choose what they will and won't pay for, so you can pay for a premium that doesn't cover your illness.

They deny coverage to people who would likely lead to a claim.

They deny claims that make it difficult, frustrating, and annoying for a physician or policyholder to be compensated.

They offer high deductibles with minimum coverage that have little value.

They write policies that make people think they are covered for illness and injuries when they aren't covered.

They will say they will pay out a higher amount than they pay.

There is no relationship between the time and materials cost and what the patient is charged.

The for-profit medical system incentivizes lawyers to file frivolous lawsuits that clog up the court system and increase the cost of health care.

Conflict of Interest

The idea of private insurance for life-saving services has conflicts of interest, which prevent effective treatment. The insurance company is supposed to pay the medical bill but must deny payment to make money. To serve the consumer's interests, the company must keep its costs low, but corporate culture pushes top dollar for corporate leaders regardless of performance. These contradictions make people do one thing and the opposite simultaneously.

30 Million Uninsured

We have a medical system that works for some and not others. Thirty million people have no health insurance in the U.S. Some put off going to a doctor until the problem becomes extreme. An illness or injury can become much worse during that time. Instead of simple preventative measures, an expensive procedure may be required. This increases the pain and suffering of the patient and requires more time, energy, and money than fixing a little problem before it becomes a big problem.

If You Are Not In a Large Group Plan, You Pay More

Insurance companies have money to hire lawyers to write contracts. If many people form a group to buy health insurance together, they can pool their money to hire a lawyer to negotiate more favorable terms. An insurance company is more willing to negotiate the terms of the contract because a lot of business is at stake. The lawyer has leverage because the insurance company knows they will lose a lot of business if they don't negotiate. Often, when individuals try to get health care, they pay much higher rates than those in a large group plan. Private individuals are no match for the negotiating power of an insurance company.

Compared to Other Countries, People in the U.S. Pay More Per Capita and Get Less Healthcare

One way to determine how our healthcare system is performing is to compare it to other countries. The Organization for Economic Co-operation and Development (OECD) compiles statistics from 32 countries. Compared to other countries, the price of medicine is much higher in the U.S. With fewer doctors and hospital beds per capita than in other countries, the demand for

doctors and hospital beds is high. In a market economy, this is a recipe for higher prices. Life expectancy is another measure of a medical system. From 1960-2010, life expectancy increased by 15 years in Japan, 11 years in OECD countries, and nine years in the U.S. **So even though we spend more money, people are dying sooner in the U.S. than in other countries.** What about the cost of medical services? In 2010, the U.S. spent $8,200 per person for health care; the next highest, Switzerland, Norway, and Netherlands, pay over $3000 less per person. The average healthcare spending for OECD countries per person per year was about $3200. So, compared to other countries, the cost of health insurance in the U.S. is quite high.

Administration, Lawsuits and Low Nutrition, High-calorie Foods Drive Up Costs

17.6% of US Gross Domestic Product (GDP) is spent on healthcare; the next highest was the Netherlands at 12%. The OECD average is 9.5%. U.S. spending is much higher for all categories of care, especially ambulatory care and administration costs. France spends $300 per person for administration costs, and the U.S. spends

$900. A hospital stay in the U.S. costs $18,000 compared to $6000 in OECD countries. The U.S. system is known for over-testing and over-treating. Doctors do this to avoid malpractice lawsuits, common in the United States and uncommon elsewhere. The for-profit law system inflates the cost of health care. Another measure of our country's health is the rate of obesity. It's higher in the United States than any other country. Just walk into most grocery stores. The stores are packed with high-calorie, low-nutrition foods. Now, 1/3 of children are overweight or obese. How do you control a system set up to make the most money it can? How do you motivate people to provide good care without charging too much money?

ObamaCare, Increase Access and Prevention,

ObamaCare was set up to make health care more accessible and more affordable. Insurance works when all the people who use the system pay into it. Since hospitals must care for people in need regardless of their ability to pay, some people use the system without paying. Inevitably, those with more resources will subsidize those with less. So healthy people will pay when they are healthy. This will build up the money required to help those who can't afford to pay. ObamaCare requires public or private insurance to provide preventative services for free. The idea is to incentivize people to get help before a small problem becomes a huge one requiring a lot of expensive medical care. Another significant change is that someone can't be denied coverage if they have an existing condition. In the past, insurance companies denied people coverage if they were sick or injured. When this happens, people wait till it's an emergency and go to the emergency room. Again, this becomes very expensive. The legislation also requires employers with over 50 employees to provide health insurance. For healthy people, the government offered lower-cost, high-deductible insurance. So, if I stay healthy, I should not need the system. When I need it, I will pay out of pocket until it hits the deductible amount, and then the health care insurance will pay. Adding many people to the system and requiring people to get health care insurance would add more people to pay. If this continues and preventative measures reduce healthcare system use, insurance prices may decrease. That's the basic idea.

Will ObamaCare work?

So, will this work? It has added millions to the healthcare system. People with existing conditions who couldn't get healthcare before were added to the system. Low-income people who couldn't afford insurance before were added to the system. Full-time workers in companies with 50 or more employees were added to the healthcare system. In 2017, around 10 million people without a government or employer health insurance plan saw the insurance price rise by 14-100%. This was done to keep up with medical costs and to make money. Some of those people can get subsidies to cover the cost increases. Others must switch insurers, which isn't so easy. Obama-Care is one more step toward single-payer, and this is what terrifies the Republicans. Some of their big-money constituents are in the health-care industry.

ObamaCare has increased the number of people insured by 24 million people, 33 million more need insurance.

People with existing conditions can't be denied service.

Now, insurance pays for prescriptions and screening.

All children get vision and dental care.

ObamaCare expanded rehabilitation, mental health, and prenatal care.

Patients in clinical trials are covered.

Potential Solutions

Increase the supply of doctors by providing government loans to students to pay for medical school. Loans would be canceled after students work two years in community health care.

Create independent review boards of qualified doctors and scientists to evaluate and censor low-performing or drug-abusing doctors and make solutions that prevent medical errors.

By sending these cases to a review board, frivolous lawsuits that clog the legal system could be avoided.

Stop drug companies from advertising and create online free reports on the performance of drugs.

Mandate government sets drug prices for the country and sets prices accordingly for companies that receive public funding for their research.

To prevent intellectual property hoarding that stops necessary research, stop granting patents on genes, cell lines, and proteins and revoke the ones that have been issued.

Ban ghostwriting drug company-sponsored articles.

So What About People Without Insurance?

If you don't have insurance, look into getting some. Look for Help; you'll find it. Ask at a public hospital or one that helps people with less money. They will help you get it. Not all government is wrong. Many people worked hard to make a system that included people with less money and resources. The system is made to help you, but you must make an effort. If your will to live is low, you must keep going. Keep in mind that many people have been depressed in their lives, and they got over it. Getting through difficulties helps you grow as a person. You can empathize and help others and realize how it enables you to reach beyond and through life's challenges. Insurance and the medical systems are set up to help you, so use it to your advantage. Like anything with a lot of power to help people, insurance and a hospital can do a lot of damage to those who need to be more informed, alert, and careful. Getting health care insurance requires significant effort for many people, so don't give up or get discouraged.

Medicare Insurance

Medicare Insurance is set up for seniors 65 or older who have paid into social security for 40 periods or 10 years. Each period is three months. Medicare used to pay for all costs, but now they are cutting back. There are Medicare Part B, C, and D, in which people pay for less necessary costs. In general, the rules keep changing, and costs keep rising. The for-profit system dominates the medical establishment. Most healthcare insurance companies are against big groups looking for healthcare coverage because it's harder to control a group with a lot of money for lawyers and negotiators. Insurance companies want to set their rates; after all, when you are bleeding to death, are you going to argue with them about whether it costs 10,000 or 1,000,000? These are complex issues. The for-profit system puts research and development money into procedures that will pay the most. This drives up costs. Until we use one system for everyone, we will all pay 20-40%

more than it should cost. This is another reason to make the most significant effort to stay out of the hospital.

Should I Get Insurance or Take a Chance and Hope for the Best

Years ago, not having health insurance was an option. As we move closer to single-payer, everyone will be included, and that will help most people. Going without health insurance is very risky. If you get sick or injured without health insurance, you could accrue considerable debt that could last a lifetime. Also, getting care may be challenging as some hospitals won't receive certain people. They may not specialize in or be set up for exceptional cases. In some medical systems, you may be their lowest priority, so you may have to wait in pain or wait till they have time or till someone is willing to help you.

On the other hand, if you are in the cash economy, you can save the money you would have paid for health insurance. Now, that may add up over time if you are very good at saving money, but if not, you may spend it on things with less value than health insurance. Now, what's more important than health insurance? Perhaps staying healthy and out of the hospital, but we can't control that. Almost all of us walk the street, work, and play in ways that expose us to risks we can't control.

Should I Stay or Should I Go

Some visit the hospital for minor aches, pains, colds, or flu. Others avoid it like the plague; some only go on their last day. Minor infections can often heal with home remedies. Muscle pains take time to heal, but a hospital visit can be avoided with pain relievers, massage, and home remedies. Some things are apparent. Extreme pain, a broken bone or out-of-joint limb, or a colossal wound requires a visit to the hospital. Some things like a stroke or heart attack may start slow and increase in pain as it gets worse. If you know the signs of these events, getting to the hospital sooner will help immensely.

What is the value of insurance?

Health insurance is a method to help people with an accident or illness requiring medical services. Without it, many people would suffer more pain and live much shorter lives. When people go to a hospital, many leave their worries about their medical condition for the hospital. I don't need to worry about my broken jaw; the doctor will take care of it. I won't have to figure out how to fix and deal with it myself. Because medical systems can save your life, they have high value. I need a house and food, but if I don't fix my body, I will die a lot sooner.

Insurance is a contract between the payer and the provider. The terms, how much is paid for what services, can be negotiated. When the government negotiates a health insurance contract, people get better service for less money. If the government runs it, it's possible to take advantage of the large numbers of people using the same system. When a large organized group governs a health care system, it's possible to maximize the benefits of the system and make it run efficiently.

Single Payer Insurance

Single-payer health care, which most developed countries have, costs less and provides more service. Often, the government sets the price for health care services. The same price is charged regardless of geography. The money comes from taxes. Since everyone is enrolled, there's a standard, simple process for getting in. You don't have to choose between companies that want your money and don't want to provide services. Doctors' education is subsidized to ensure enough doctors are available to do public service or pay out of pocket for their education.

10 Reasons for Single Payer

1. Reduce pain and suffering while improving the quality of life.

When everyone is included in the medical system, we have a more fair, equitable, and just medical system that provides necessary services that reduce the pain, suffering, and loss of millions of people.

2. Pay less and get more back.

Single-payer is the most cost-efficient way to provide healthcare. Countries with single payers have better healthcare for less money.

3. Spreading risk

If 300 million people enroll in one system, the risk is shared. People pay into the system until they are sick or injured. They pay what they can and take what they need. This matters less when premiums are affordable. The benefit for healthy people is knowing they are covered if they are sick or injured. In the for-profit medical system, they pay high premiums anyway, or some don't get insurance and risk owing significant amounts of money to pay for medical services. When people know they have health care, they have less stress and can prevent going to the hospital again.

4. More Money to Spend

If done correctly, a single-payer system would reduce the money spent on healthcare. People would have more money in their pockets to spend on other things.

5. Frivolous Lawsuits Clog the Judicial System

The for-profit medical system incentivizes lawyers to file frivolous lawsuits that clog up the court system and increase the cost of health care.

6. Performance Controls Reduce the Number of Bad Doctors and Reduce Mistakes

A government-run healthcare system could compile statistics on what procedures work and which don't, which doctors perform well, and which doctors are better off doing something else. With these quality and performance controls in place, we would get better care for less money.

7. Keep Your Healthcare Regardless of Your Job

If you lose or change your job, you still have health insurance.

8. Single Payer is More Efficient

Expensive health care reduces our competitive advantage with other countries that spend less and get more for their health care money. An efficient health care system makes a country more competitive and results in fewer people taking off work, fewer people taking time to find an insurance company, and less frustration and agony trying to get an insurance company to do what they are supposed to.

9. Universal Enrollment

Single-payer requires all or most people to participate in the single-payer system. This ensures a large enough group of people to share the risk. When one person is sick, many others are paying. This spreads out the risk. When enough people are enrolled, and the system prevents mistakes and corruption, all people have healthcare, and premiums aren't excessive. With one option, the single-payer system, people don't have to choose between this or that insurance. They know they are covered. It's similar to social security.

10. Reduce administration costs.

Medicare uses about 3% of its budget for administration costs; for profit healthcare system costs can be many times higher.

Facts from 2010 from the Organization for Economic Co-operation and Development (OECD) — an international economic group comprised of 34 member nations:

The U.S. has fewer doctors per capita than other countries.

The U.S. has 2.7 doctors per 1000 patients, and OECD has 3.4 per 1000.

U.S. has 2.6 hospital beds per 1000, compared to 3.4 per 1000 for OECD

From 1960-2010, life expectancy increased by 15 years in Japan, 11 years in OECD countries, and only nine years in the U.S.

In 2010, the U.S. spent 8,200 per person for health care; next highest, Switzerland, Norway, and the Netherlands spent over $3000 less per person

The average healthcare spending for OECD countries per person per year was about $3200.

17.6% of the US Gross Domestic Product (GDP) is spent on healthcare; the next highest was the Netherlands at 12%; the OECD average is 9.5%

U.S. spending is much higher for all categories of care, especially ambulatory care and administration costs

France spends $300 per person for administration costs, and the U.S. spends $900

A hospital stay in the U.S. costs $18000 compared to $6000 in OECD countries' U.S. system is known for over-testing and over-treating

1/3 of children are overweight or obese.

Obesity rates in the U.S. are highest in the U.S. over the past 20 years.

CHAPTER 9
HERBS

Herbs

Our bodies require peak nutrition to maximize mental and physical performance. Whole foods and herbs offer many vitamins, minerals, and compounds that may prevent heart disease, stroke, and diabetes. Herbs empower your body to resist infection, heal when sick, and build up your body's power. Some make you feel and look 10-30 years younger (Sarsaparilla Root). Herbs remove toxins that prevent you from realizing your goals. Herbs contain compounds too unique to be replicated by big pharmaceutical companies. Many herbs are beneficial with few side effects. Some plants and herbs will kill you. Getting to know and use herbs can enhance your body and mind for peak performance, which can help you stay out of the hospital.

Herbs offer the following benefits:

Empower the immune system to fight infections and diseases.

Deliver integrated nutrition with vitamins, minerals, and compounds.

Reduce inflammation by killing and removing toxins, bacteria, and viruses.

Enhance your mental and physical performance.

Prevent cancer, heart disease and diabetes.

Improve the quality and strength of bones, muscles, veins, blood, organs, and brain.

Many herbs have few side effects, but consult a doctor before taking them.

People don't use herbs because:

They need more time or desire to make tea, take tinctures, and do research.

Some people don't like the taste of herbs.

They need an herbalist, books, or the internet to help them figure out how to use the herbs.

They need the money or knowledge required to use herbs.

Herbs for Detox

It's nearly impossible to stop toxins from entering your body. Even a pristine wilderness contains pollution from the wind, water, people, and animals. Food may have pesticides, herbicides, and fertilizers that can make you sick. On the job, many workers are exposed to chemicals and vapors that can wreak havoc in the body. Indoor air pollution is many times higher than outside. Of course, it's best to prevent exposure, but somehow, it gets in, so how do you get it out? Here are some ways to detox:

I will eat as much raw food per day as I can. I will chew it and swallow. I will drink at least 8 cups of water per day.

I will research detox herbs and find one to focus on each week or month.

I will do aerobic exercises at least every other day.

I will always eat at least two fresh fruits or vegetables with my meals.

Pharmaceutical Drugs

Drugs are extracted from herbs, animals, fungi, and natural compounds. They are derivatives of what occurs in nature. Medicines are stripped from nature and may create an unbalanced impact on the body. Some drugs have significant side effects. Most drugs have yet to stand the test of herbs. Herbs have been written about and tested by people for thousands of years. Herbs often have fewer side effects than drugs. Some contain hundreds of compounds with multiple effects.

These may balance the body and reduce the intensity of side effects. The advantage of drugs is that they can be used for specific applications. Be careful to read about the side effects of your medicines.

Herbs for Energy

With potent compounds to boost your energy, herbs like Ginseng, Sarsaparilla Root, and Suma Root invigorate your life. Energy herbs grow your desire to be physically and mentally active. Unique compounds increase metabolism, burn fat, add muscle, and boost immunity. I've used Sarsaparilla root to give me the courage and power to get beyond feeling weak, stuck, and unmotivated. With sterol-like compounds, Sarsaparilla Root removes inhibitions, increases physical and mental energy, and helps you move beyond limitations. Native people use Sarsaparilla Root to stop Syphilis. These get-up-and-go herbs can maximize physical and mental performance and boost your immune system.

Researching on the Internet

The internet is a vast resource for learning how to use herbs to heal. In a search engine, type in herbs and the desired outcome. So, in the Google search box, I type "herbs immune system," "herbs headache," "herbs detox," "herbs wisdom," or "herbs happiness." When you do this, a large number of results come up. Many websites provide information on growing, using, and storing herbs. Make a little hobby out of this and have fun growing, using, and storing herbs.

Herbs for Immunity

If you learn to boost your immune system, you can fight infections that put you in the hospital. Herbs like echinacea, garlic, and Siberian ginseng grow your immune system. Learn to use them when feeling weak, tired, and sick. If you feel your throat getting too dry or aches and pain in your body, or if you have a red, swollen, and painful sore, it's time to take action. At the first signs, get rest and start taking these herbs to give your body the power to build up your immune system. Take the immune-building herbs, echinacea, garlic, and ginseng. Make tea, take a tincture, or eat the powder. Some herbs, like an Echinacea tincture, will go to work immediately. Others, like Siberian ginseng, can take months to get the maximum effect. If you have a sore that won't heal, make a poultice and apply it, and it's like your infection will recede.

Herbs for the Lymph system

The lymph system goes to work at the first stages of an illness or infection. It's a network of tissues and organs that removes toxins and supplies white blood cells. Inflammation occurs when white blood cells attack a bacteria, virus, or toxin. As your body swells, toxins accumulate. Herbs like burdock, dandelion, and lobelia can help remove toxins, keep the swelling down, and help you concentrate. As toxins accumulate, your thinking may be impaired. Taking these herbs once or twice for two days to 2 weeks can be a good cleansing routine. Some that are mild may be taken frequently. These herbs improve digestion and skin problems and boost your energy.

Herbs to Combat Infections

Infections kill many people each year. As antibiotics are overused, bacteria and viruses overcome the medicine and kill people. With effort, you can learn to use herbs to minimize infections. Herbs may be used internally and externally to fight infections. Make a tea or tincture for internal use. Use a poultice, salve, or simple clay mix eternally. A poultice can be made from many different plants and will suck out the poison and increase the speed of healing. Herbs may be used in a variety of ways. One way to get rid of athletes' feet is to heat green tea leaves and cover the whole area of the fungus. Then, cover it with a plastic bag and a sock, and the problem will be gone in the morning. This may last weeks or months as the tea seeps deep into your foot. French Green Clay will quickly improve your skin as it sucks out the poison. Wild plantain, with astringent properties, pulls out toxins and rejuvenates the skin. Choose what works best for you. Using both methods may produce the best results. You can use herbs to build up your immune system slowly. This may take months, but it is good to do when you think your stress levels will rise when you have the time or to prepare to maximize your physical and mental performance. In the winter, Siberian ginseng will help your body adapt to the cold. It will stop your fear of the cold and stop your shivering.

Herbs for Physical Performance

If you want your body to perform well under pressure, give it nutrition to go faster, harder, and longer. Think about your body, bones, blood, muscles, nerves, and hormones. All perform special functions requiring vitamins, minerals, and compounds to live well. What if your bones are weak because they don't have enough calcium, your blood doesn't have enough iron, and your nerves are fried from too much coffee? These things can slow you down in a big way. Peak nutrition maximizes different nutrition sources. Athletes looking for advantages turn to Siberian ginseng, sarsaparilla root, and other herbs. These boost metabolism, increase testosterone, and build muscle power. Alfalfa is rich in chlorophyll, minerals, and vitamins A, B, D, and K. Drinking a tea rich in nutrients helps you stay healthy and strong, and will make your hair grow like a weed.

Peak Nutrition

To get peak nutrition, increase the range and quality of your food sources. With more food sources, you will provide your body with a wide range of minerals, vitamins, and compounds to build the strength of your bones and muscles while improving your immune system. Wild plants, homegrown food, food from farmers, and organic food can increase the different food sources. Harvesting, drying, and using wild foods is another source of nutrition. With effort, you can learn how to identify and use these plants to improve nutrition. Herbs are another source of nutrition. With many different compounds from different parts of plants, herbs offer a vast range of vitamins, minerals, and unique compounds to empower your performance. Supplements provide another range of nutrition but are not plants and are not alive, but may offer specific benefits to improve your health. You can build your body's physical and mental power with diverse food sources.

Monoculture

Supermarket food is produced through monoculture and petrochemical farming. Monoculture, one plant per field, is a standard method of agriculture that uses gasoline for tractors and herbicides, pesticides, and fertilizers to make the plants grow. All weeds are eliminated with cultivation and chemicals. Pesticides, herbicides, and fertilizers may be in the food. Residue from mechanical processes may also enter the food. The more it is processed, the less value it has. Imagine what happens to a piece of grain. It's pulverized, mixed, and baked.

After that, it is packaged inside a paper or plastic wrapper. It is transported to the store, where it may sit for a day to a couple of weeks before you eat it. Now compare that to walking outside, picking and eating some chives. Imagine how the chives enter and energize your body. The chives have lasted the whole winter without any coddling or processing. They rise strong out of the ground in early spring. They grow well in 60-degree temperatures. The bright color radiates life. The point is that the quality of familiar food, including fruits and vegetables, is challenging to determine and is often lower quality than less processed, organic, or wild food. If you want to stay out of the hospital, diversify your food sources; grow your food, buy from a farmer, and learn how to harvest and eat wild food.

Herbs for Mental Acuity

Build your body to build your brain. Herbs provide peak nutrition to help your brain perform at the highest level. Your brain requires circulation to small nerves and tissues to function well. Gingko and gotu-kola increase blood vessel strength and resilience while increasing blood flow to the brain. Ginseng and rosemary improve cognitive function. Using herbs regularly to keep your brain functioning at a high level will pay big dividends in the long run.

Functions of Herbs

Herbs are classified according to function. Aromatics contain volatile oils that act on different systems of the body. Adaptogens balance and strengthen your whole body more than one organ. Calming herbs feed the nerves, reduce tension, and avoid circular thinking. Different herbs have similar functions. Damiana, rose and vanilla are aphrodisiacs. Herbs affect people in different ways. One person may like the action of rose, but not damiana. You may choose an herb for its taste, how it grows or how it effects you. As you learn more about herbs, you can select the ones you like to use and experiment with others.

Combining Herbs

By combining herbs, you can design high-impact teas. Essiac tea, a combination of burdock, sheep sorrel, slippery elm, and Indian rhubarb, is used against cancer. However, scientific studies do not confirm this. You can take recipes and add other teas as you experiment with what works and doesn't work. Happy tea is a recipe I made to maximize mental and physical performance. It uses alfalfa, oat straw, ginkgo, gotu-kola, lemon balm, passion flower, and damiana to provide peak nutrition for the whole body. Curry is considered a spice but has herbs that function like medicine. You can develop your recipes as you research and find plants that fascinate you for different reasons.

Marijuana

Marijuana generates positive consequences, including:

It helps reduce stress and negative feelings.

Reduce depression by making you feel high and forget negative thinking.

It helps you get a long and deep sleep.

It may increase your physical energy and sex drive.

It may help with epilepsy and nerve problems.

It helps you forget difficult people and painful memories.

Increases your appetite.

It may help you deal with difficult people by allowing you to forget abuse and focus on other things.

It may reduce nausea and boredom.

Marijuana has negative consequences, including:

It reduces short-term memory.

It increases appetite.

Some people get paranoid, feel disoriented, and lose their sense of self.

It may not be suitable for driving or using heavy machinery.

It may increase heart rate and trigger a heart attack or stroke.

In 2018, marijuana is legal in some states and illegal in others. Often, people have to get it from a clandestine source, which may generate several problems. You can get arrested and face severe consequences in some states. It's not clear how potent marijuana is until you try it. In general, the potency of marijuana has increased. For some people, one puff is too much. It can increase your heart rate, make you feel disoriented, and make you forget what you are doing. So why get stoned? Getting stoned is a release from the world's stress, reduces pain, helps you forget annoying people, and may give you physical and mental energy to get work done. Because it is so complex and different varieties have different effects, you may be unable to predict how it will affect you. It may or may not help you get work done. Some people don't like being around people who are stoned. It may change your personality. Marijuana can make you happy or high, and this can prevent depression. For some, it helps them focus and inspires them to play or practice music. Because it has been illegal, marijuana has given birth to a counterculture. Some enjoy it, but that may change as it becomes more accepted. Derivatives of marijuana have helped people cope with extreme nerve-related problems. It makes them settle down and relax instead of having convulsions. Can it keep you out of the hospital? If you use it correctly, yes, it can help you live a whole and prosperous life, but some marijuana will hinder your ability to drive a car or do dangerous things. It can also help. This is a powerful herb, and, like many others, use it with caution.

CHAPTER 10
HOSPITAL STRATEGIES

I f you get sticker shock in an airport movie theater or baseball game, a hospital could be many times worse. They don't put a price tag on their services. They do them, and you are charged later. Sometimes, insurance will cover the charges, and sometimes, not. Do you have to call every time you use the bathroom? Ask your insurance company and the nurse, doctor, and administrator. If you have no money, tell them. They could do the minimum. It's a loaded institution. The stakes are high, and when you are weak and sick or injured, it can be impossible to prevent people from taking advantage of you or just doing things that may bring financial ruin and leave you bankrupt or feeling like an indentured servant. Generally, take care of yourself as much as possible and avoid using anything that may cost a lot of money at a hospital.

Sometimes, you don't have a choice; you must go in. Try to have someone ready to be your advocate before you go in. Make sure you avoid these mistakes:

Private rooms cost extra and may not be covered by insurance. Let them know as soon as possible that you don't need a private room. Non-private rooms mean you are put in a room with another person.

You are separated from that person by a curtain. Since your stay may be shorter, most people can live with another person for a few days.

If in the emergency room, remember you are an outpatient until formally admitted and then an inpatient. Outpatients pay more for tests, x-rays, and supplies. Generally, they can hold you for two midnights before you are officially accepted. Sometimes, it's hard to know if you need the tests. If you feel reasonably good, similar to normal, then it's ok to skip some of the tests. Do self-tests to see how well you can function.

Ask all unknown visitors to your bedside who sent them and what they are doing. Sometimes, doctors, nurses, or specialists who do very little work for a lot of money will show up. People have been charged over $500 for these visits. Try to get a sense of what is needed. As the doctor says, if you are slowly progressing, you don't need that much attention from another medical person.

You may be asked if you want special hospital equipment. Suppose it doesn't seem critical or seems like something you could do without or get one yourself; refuse it. These will increase your premium and take up space in your closet later.

Quick Points

-Avoid private rooms.

-Avoid out-of-network care. Pay copay and deductibles, not out-of-network care.

-Avoid outpatient emergency services like tests, x-rays, and unnecessary procedures.

-Track all people who come to your hospital bedside.

-Refuse equipment you don't need or can supply yourself.

Generally, take care of yourself as much as possible and learn to do self-tests. Can I see, hear, taste, smell, eat, sleep, pee, poop, and exercise like normal. If not, where is the pain, and what is the goal? I want my tooth pulled to stop the infection. I like the pain in my leg to stop so I can walk. I need to control the disease so I have the energy to do my work. Be firm with doctors and nurses. Discuss the risk of not doing specific tests, procedures, and medications. Can I do those things later if my situation gets worse? If there's no chance or low chance of getting better, let them know if all you want are some painkillers or maybe nothing at all. Some people don't like how drugs distort pain. You lose the cues your body is sending you. I assume you will get billed for all care unless your provider says it's covered.

ABOUT THE AUTHOR

Dan Paul grew up in Lake Wobegon fishing, playing sports and building houses. After attending the University of Wisconsin, Madison and working at the linear fusion reactor lab, he explored alternatives to the dominant codes. While staying in coops, communes, and squats around the country, he learned the fundamentals of setting up and operating progressive, radical and sustainable alternatives to the codes corporations and nations.

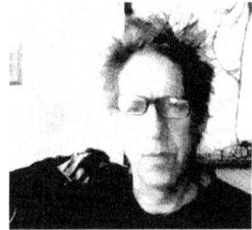

f X ⊙

ALSO BY DAN PAUL

Philosophy of Action Design and Multiplicity by Dan Paul

Book 1 Auto Free Design

Book 2 Workers Health Handbook

Book 3 Save Your Life Prevent Hospital Use

Book 4 Coop Owners Handbook

Book 5 Eye on AI Meeting Needs Sustainably

Book 6 Travels on the Nomadic Terrain

Book 7 Tales of the Urban Shaman

Book 8 Housing in the Danger Zone

Book 9 Corona Time

Book 10 Philosophy of Design, Action and Multiplicity

Coming soon;

Landlords Against Eviction

Auto Free USA

Websites

https://viaradmedia.org

https://autofreedesign.com

http://workershealthhandbook.com

http://sylphu.com

www.ingramcontent.com/pod-product-compliance
Lightning Source LLC
Chambersburg PA
CBHW060518280326
41933CB00014B/3021

* 9 7 8 1 9 5 3 1 0 4 0 5 2 *